Mistletoe

V.K. Roberts

ISBN 978-1-0980-3353-8 (paperback)
ISBN 978-1-0980-3354-5 (digital)

Copyright © 2020 by V.K. Roberts

All rights reserved. No part of this publication may be reproduced, distributed, or transmitted in any form or by any means, including photocopying, recording, or other electronic or mechanical methods without the prior written permission of the publisher. For permission requests, solicit the publisher via the address below.

Christian Faith Publishing, Inc.
832 Park Avenue
Meadville, PA 16335
www.christianfaithpublishing.com

Printed in the United States of America

I dedicate this book to my wife, children, grandchildren, and great-grandchildren now and in the future.

Readers Guide

This is an interactive children's book. Using different inflections in your voice as you read each page would be an experience for the child.

For example, use a deep voice describing the *big* toe or a sad voice describing the *middle* toe.

Also interact with the child as you touch each toe by emphasizing what the words describe (i.e., "tickle," "wiggle," "ouch").

The book will begin in the middle. You can start on the left foot Page 16 or right foot Page 17.

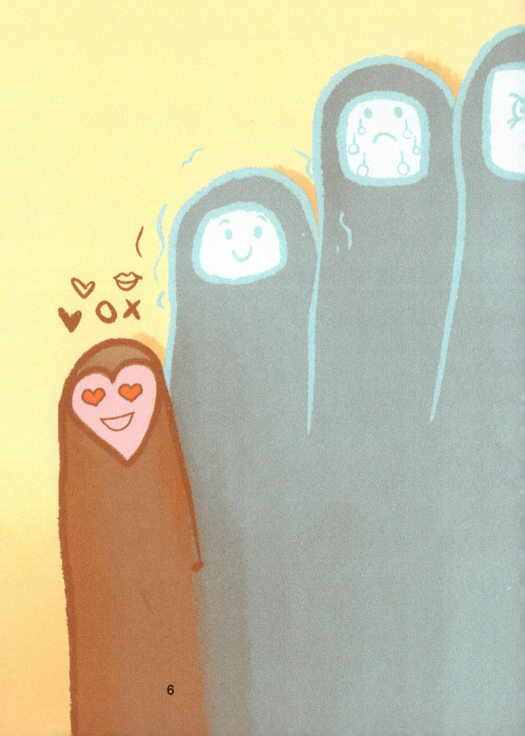

I may be small and at the end but

I am filled with love and "KISSES"

From the top of my head all the

way down to me... "MISTLETOE"!!!!!

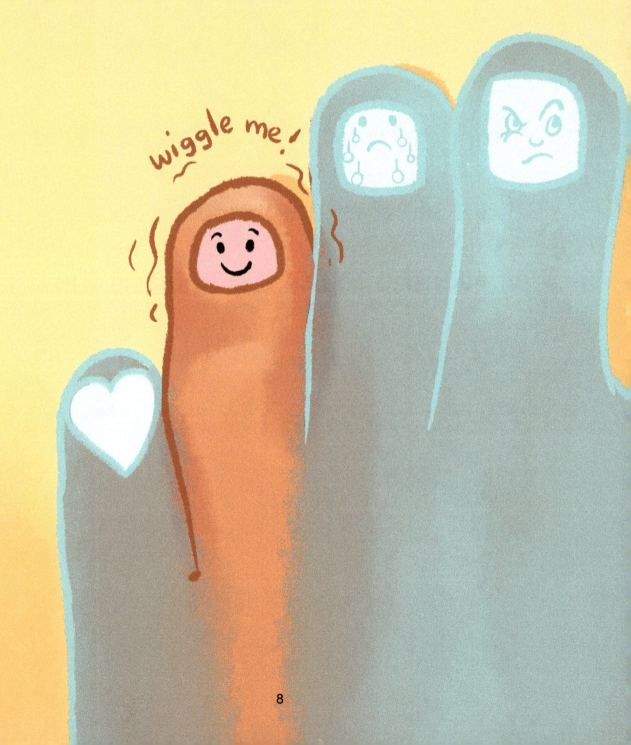

Call me "TICKLE" toe!

Just give me a "WIGGLE" and

I will just giggle and giggle!

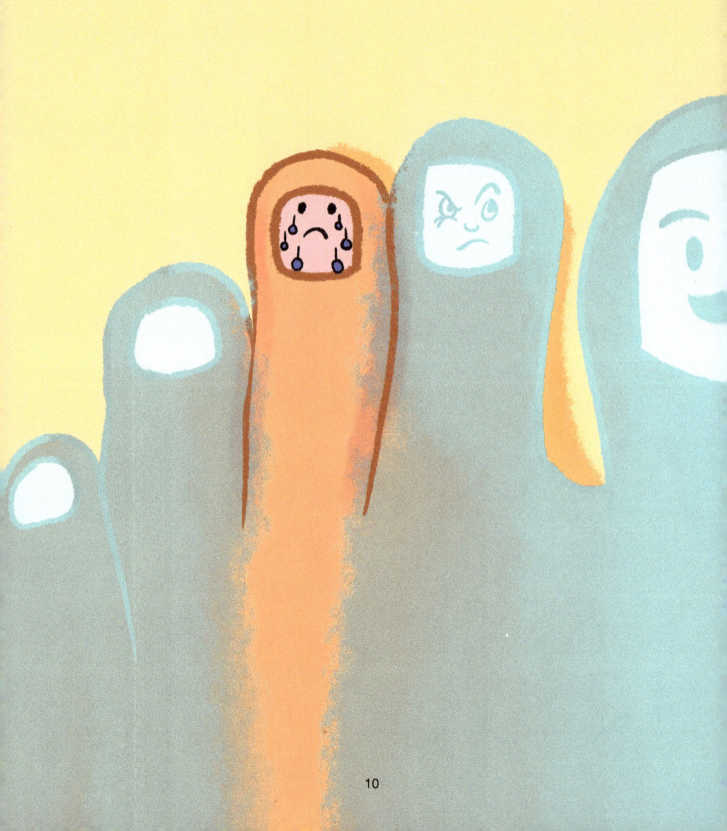

I am in the middle but do not have a name... BOO! HOO! Please give me one since I am a part of YOU!!

Now I am ready to Go! Go! Go!

I am happy now! My name is ☐ toe.

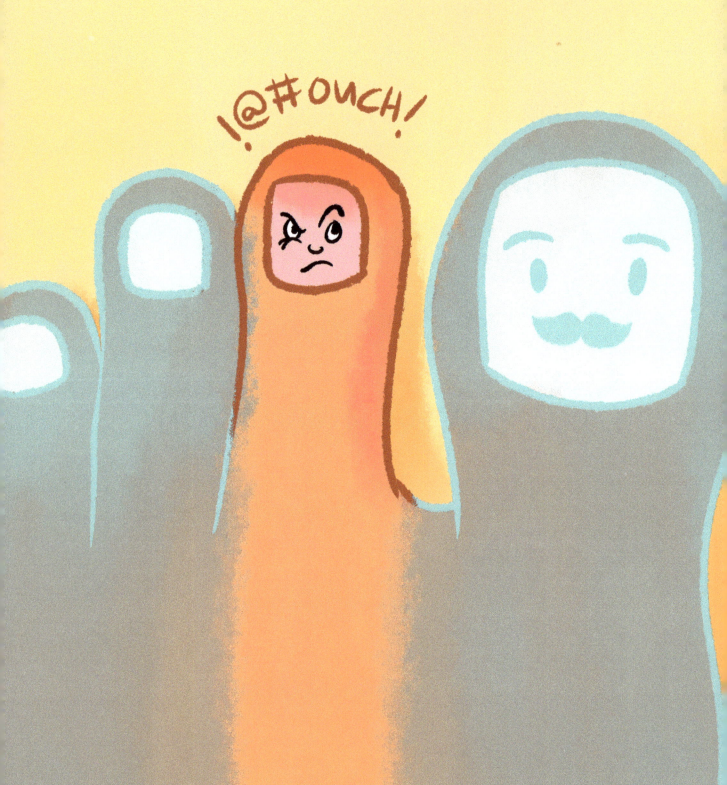

¡Hola!! My name is "STUB" toe!

When it is dark at night,

I find the edge of the couch and

I must yell "OUCH"!!!!

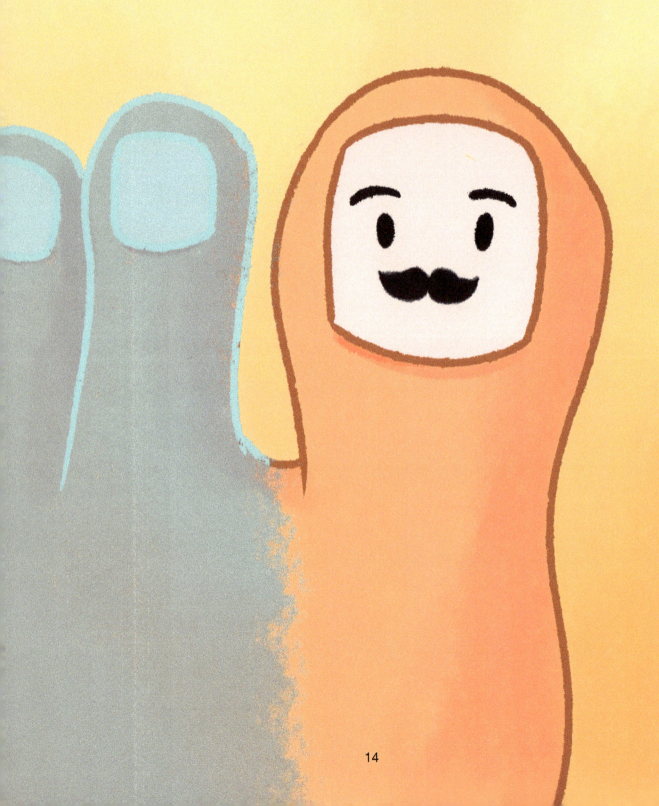

Hi!! I'm "BIG" toe!

I help you grow big and tall

And let you walk straight

so you don't *FALL*.

Left Foot ←

Right Foot

→

Hi!! I'm "BIG" toe!

I help you grow big and tall

And let you walk straight

so you don't *FALL*.

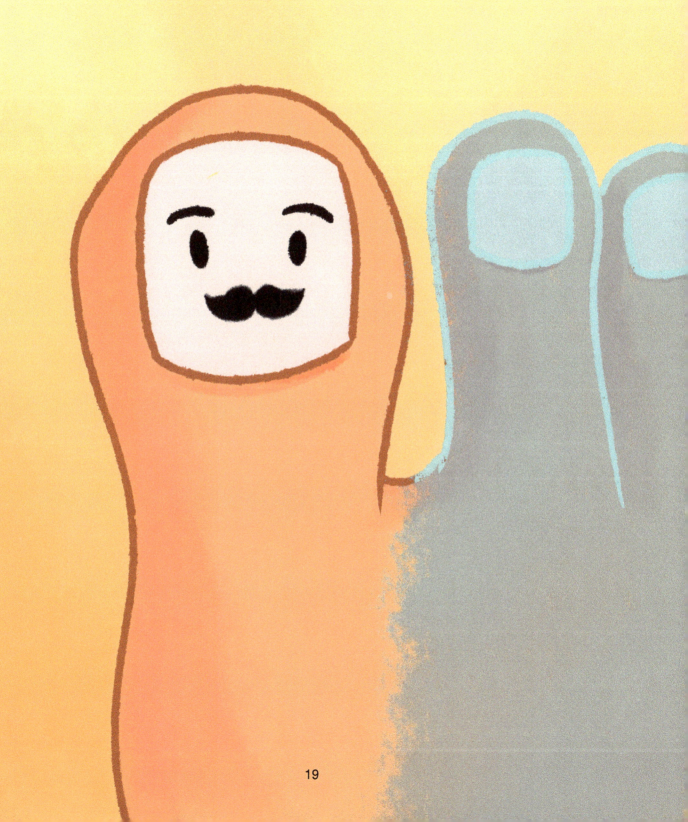

¡Hola!! My name is "STUB" toe!

When it is dark at night,

I find the edge of the couch and

I must yell "OUCH"!!!!

!@#OUCH!

I am in the middle but do

not have a name... BOO! HOO!

Please give me one since

I am a part of YOU!!

I am happy now! My name is _____ toe.

Now I am ready to Go! Go! Go!

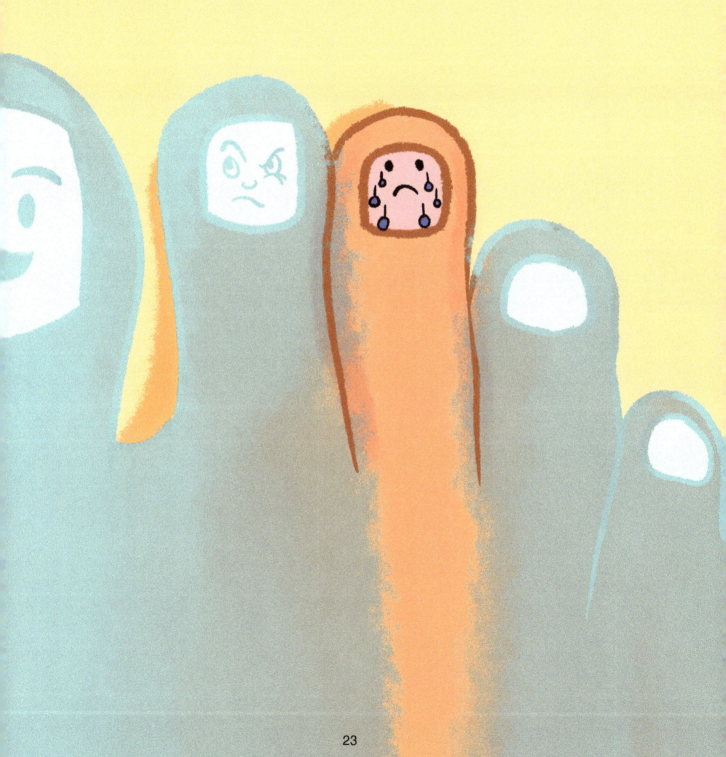

Call me "TICKLE" toe!

Just give me a "WIGGLE" and

I will just giggle and giggle!

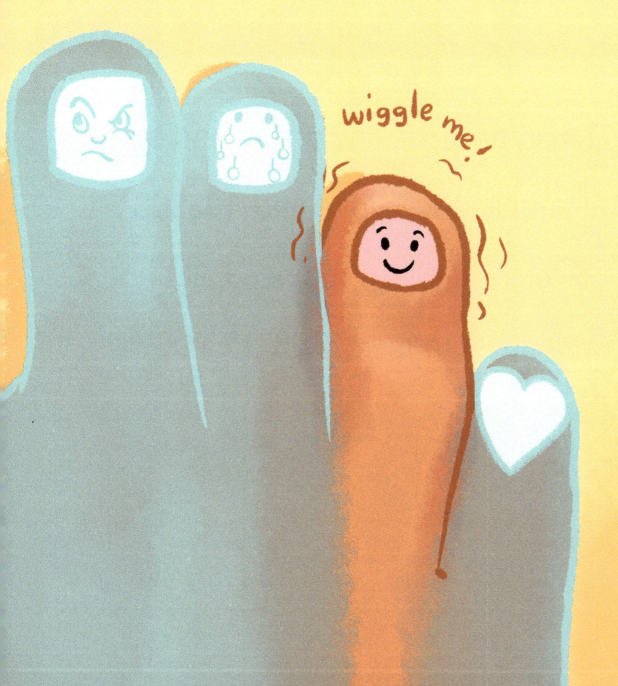

I may be small and at the end but

I am filled with love and "KISSES"

From the top of my head all the

way down to me… "MISTLETOE"!!!!!

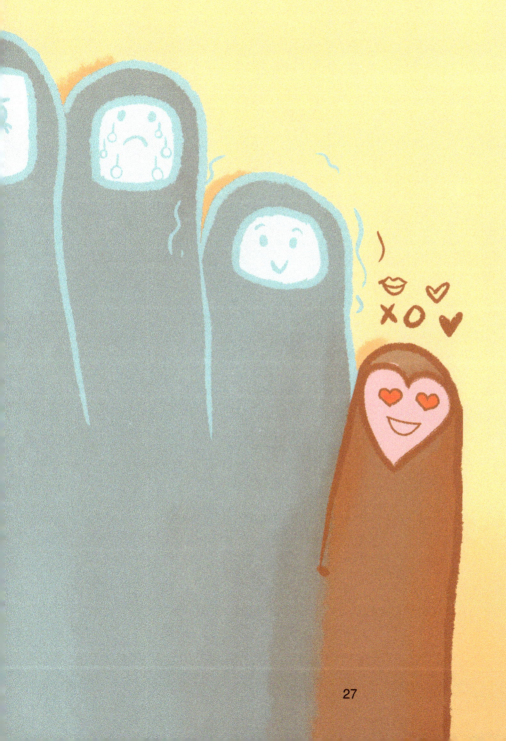

About the Author

I wrote this book using the name V. K. Roberts. The "V" honors my daughter Victoria, the "K" honors my daughter Kimberlee and Robert is my first name. I hope you have fond memories reading this book to a young child.

CPSIA information can be obtained
at www.ICGtesting.com
Printed in the USA
LVHW021459080121
675967LV00006B/217